THE MAGNET VISION

Magnet organizations will serve as the fount of knowledge and expertise for the delivery of nursing care globally. They will be solidly grounded in core Magnet principles, flexible, and constantly striving for discovery and innovation. They will lead the reformation of health care; the discipline of nursing; and care of the patient, family, and community.

THE COMMISSION ON MAGNET RECOGNITION, 2008

American Nurses Credentialing Center

As the largest and most prestigious nurse credentialing organization in the United States, the American Nurses Credentialing Center (ANCC) provides individuals and organizations in the nursing profession with the tools they need on their journey to excellence. ANCC recognizes healthcare organizations for nursing excellence through the Magnet Recognition Program®.

Commission on Magnet

The ANCC's Commission on Magnet Recognition (COM) is a voluntary governing body that oversees the Magnet Recognition Program. COM members are appointed by the ANCC's Board of Directors and include representatives from various sectors of the nursing community—executive leaders, nurse managers, staff nurses, long-term-care nurses, advanced-practice nurses (APRNs)—as well as one member representing the public. The COM makes the final determination to award Magnet™ designation.

Magnet Appraisers

Appraisers are leading expert nurses with demonstrated proficiency and experience in various organizational and specialty backgrounds relevant to the Magnet Recognition Program. Appraisers are selected through a competitive application process and undergo intensive training in the interpretation and evaluation of Sources of Evidence before assignment to any appraiser team. They assess applicant documents, conduct site visits, and prepare the final report to the COM.

Magnet Program Office

The ANCC's Magnet Program Office staff manage and coordinate all aspects of the application and appraisal process. Contact information is available at **www.nursecredentialing.org/magnet.**

Published by American Nurses Credentialing Center
8515 Georgia Avenue
Silver Spring, MD 20910-3492

© 2011 by American Nurses Credentialing Center, Silver Spring, MD
Second Edition Printed July 2011

The American Nurses Credentialing Center (ANCC) is a subsidiary of the American Nurses Association (ANA).

Disclaimer

Please note: this is an abridged version of the Magnet Recognition Program Application Manual. If your organization is considering pursuing Magnet recognition, the 2008 edition of the Magnet Manual is essential for understanding the full scope of application requirements. It is the only authorized publication that provides detailed information on the instructions and process for documentation submission. To order a copy of the 2008 Magnet Manual, or obtain additional information about the Magnet Recognition Program, visit our web site at **www.nursecredentialing.org/magnet**.

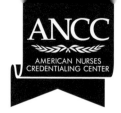

THE MAGNET MODEL COMPONENTS AND SOURCES OF EVIDENCE
Magnet Recognition Program®

TABLE OF CONTENTS

Preface

ANCC's Magnet Recognition Program was developed to recognize healthcare organizations that provide excellence in nursing practice. The number of institutions credentialed through this process continues to climb. A sizable body of research provides evidence that Magnet hospitals do make a difference. As we move forward into the 21st century, a global nursing shortage, aging population, and technologic advances pose challenges that require reformation in healthcare delivery. Magnet hospitals are poised to lead the way with outstanding quality and professionalism.

As a result, a growing number of sectors in the healthcare community have expressed interest in learning more about the characteristics of a Magnet environment. *The Magnet Model Components and Sources of Evidence* is our response to this request. It is an abridged version of the Magnet Recognition Program Application Manual and includes key program elements: the Magnet Model and its components; the Sources of Evidence used in the appraisal process; and a discussion of the increasing focus on outcomes.

It is our hope that this introductory guide will serve as a resource to those who seek to understand the important variables that interact to create a culture of excellence—one that attracts and retains highly skilled nurses who provide exemplary professional practice, create new knowledge, and impact quality outcomes.

Karen Drenkard, PhD, RN, NEA-BC, FAAN
Director, Magnet Recognition Program®
American Nurses Credentialing Center

1

The Magnet Model

The Forces of Magnetism™ (FOM) that were identified more than 25 years ago have remained remarkably stable—a testament to their enduring value. The Magnet Recognition Program has developed and evolved over time in response to changes in the healthcare environment.

STATISTICAL FOUNDATION— THE EMPIRICAL MODEL

In 2007, the ANCC commissioned a statistical analysis of final appraisal scores for applicants under the 2005 Magnet Recognition Program Application Manual (ANCC, 2004). The project goal was to examine the relationships among the FOM by investigating alternative frameworks for structuring the Sources of Evidence and inform development of the new Magnet Model. This newly-emerged Model would provide a fresh perspective on the Sources of Evidence and how they interplay to create a work environment that supports excellence in nursing practice.

Using a combination of factor analysis, cluster analysis, and multi-dimensional scaling, final Source of Evidence scores were examined to determine how they might be organized based solely on their empirical properties. The results suggested an alternative framework for grouping the Sources of Evidence, collapsing them into fewer domains than the 14 FOMs. The empiric model yielded from this analysis informed the conceptual development of the new Magnet Model (see Figure 1).

FIGURE 1. MAGNET MODEL

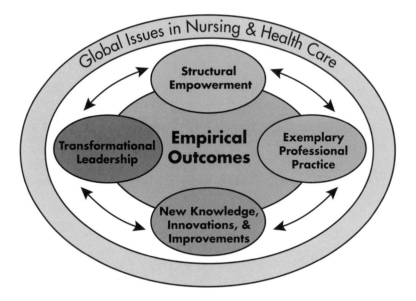

In 2007, with input from a broad representation of stakeholders, the COM developed a Model for Magnet that reflected current research on organizational behavior. This Model guides the transition of Magnet principles to focus healthcare organizations on achieving superior performance as evidenced by outcomes. Evidence-based practice, innovation, evolving technology, and patient partnerships are all evident in the Model.

TABLE 1. DERIVATION OF THE MAGNET MODEL

FORCES OF MAGNETISM	EMPIRICAL DOMAINS OF EVIDENCE	MAGNET MODEL COMPONENTS
Quality of Nursing Leadership Management Style	Leadership	Transformational Leadership
Organizational Structure Personnel Policies and Programs Community and the Healthcare Organization Image of Nursing Professional Development	Resource Utilization and Development	Structural Empowerment
Professional Models of Care Consultation and Resources Autonomy Nurses as Teachers Interdisciplinary Relations Quality of Care: Ethics, Patient Safety, and Quality Infrastructure Quality Improvement	Professional Practice Model Safe and Ethical Practice Autonomous Practice Quality Processes	Exemplary Professional Practice
Quality of Care: Research and Evidence-Based Practice Quality Improvement	Research	New Knowledge, Innovations, and Improvements
Quality of Care	Outcomes	Empirical Quality Outcomes

The FOM are still valid, but the concepts contained within them can be viewed from the perspective of the five Model components. See Table 1, above, for the relationships among the FOM, the empiric domains of evidence, and the Magnet Model components. See Appendix A for a description of the FOM.

FOCUS ON OUTCOMES

Previous Magnet application manuals emphasized structure and process. Although structure and process create the infrastructure for excellence, the outcomes of that infrastructure are essential to a culture of excellence and innovation.

Simple definitions are set forth to differentiate among structure, process, and outcomes:
- **Structure** is defined as the characteristics of the organization and the healthcare system, including leadership, availability of resources, and professional practice models.
- **Process** is defined as the actions involving the delivery of nursing and healthcare services to patients, including practices that are safe and ethical, autonomous, and evidence based, with efforts focused on quality improvement.
- **Outcomes** are defined as quantitative and qualitative evidence related to the impact of structure and process on the patient, nursing workforce, organization, and consumer. These outcomes are dynamic and measurable and may be reported at an individual unit, department, population, or organizational level.

Examples of empirical quality outcomes are listed below.

Patient Outcomes
- Risk-adjusted mortality index
- Healthcare-acquired infections
- Falls and injuries associated with falls
- Hospital-acquired pressure ulcer occurrence/prevalence
- Patient overall satisfaction
- Patient satisfaction with nursing care
- Patient satisfaction with educational information

- Patient satisfaction with pain management
- Patient perception of safety
- Specialty population-specific outcomes

Nurse Outcomes
- Level of nurse engagement
- Level of nurse satisfaction
- Perception of nurse autonomy
- Turnover and vacancy rates
- Percentage of direct-care registered nurses (RNs) with certification
- Percentage of nurse leaders with certification
- Educational preparation of staff
- Rates and types of staff injuries
- Staff perception of safe culture and work environment
- Staff perception of orientation and/or effectiveness of continuing education programs

Organizational Outcomes
- Efficiency and/or elimination of waste
- Chief nursing officer (CNO) impact on system-level change

Consumer Outcomes
- Impact of community outreach programs
- Community health and welfare

2

Organizational Overview

The following documents must be present for the appraisers to score the Sources of Evidence. The Sources of Evidence that correlate with an Organizational Overview item for scoring are indicated in parentheses following the item. See the web site at **www.nursecredentialing.org/ Magnet/Magnet-TablesTemplates.aspx** for required tables.

Contextual Information

1. A description of the applicant organization in terms of:
   - Mission
   - Vision
   - Values
   - History
   - Geographical location
   - Services provided
   - Number of licensed beds
   - Total RN full-time equivalents
   - Population(s) served

Include an ethnic profile of the nursing staff, client population, and community served.

2. The current chief nursing officer's (CNO) job description and curriculum vitae.

Transformational Leadership

3. Copies of the most recent annual reports and quality and strategic plans for the organization and nursing services. These can be formal documents or less formal methods used to inform the staff of activities related to the strategic plan. (TL1)

4. A budget summary for the most recent fiscal year, actual to budget, for nursing education, conference attendance, and research. (TL2 & EP12)

5. The administrative and nursing organizational chart(s). Describe the CNO's structural and operational relationships to all areas in which nursing is practiced. (TL4)

6. A table of nurse executives, nurse managers, and supervisors and their:
   * Credentials;
   * Earned professional certification(s);
   * Professional organization memberships, activities, and offices held; and
   * Professional development programs and formal academic education attended during the 24 months prior to documentation submission. (TL6)

Structural Empowerment

7. A table that displays direct-care nurses' participation in professional organizations/associations and activities at the local, state, national, and/or international levels. Include office(s) held. (SE2)

8. The policies and procedures that govern/guide professional development programs, such as tuition reimbursement; access to web-based education; and participation in local, regional, national, and international conferences/meetings. (SE3, SE4, & SE5)

9. The assessment for the continuing education needs for nurses at all levels and settings and the related implementation plan. (SE5)

10. A list of the continuing education programs (classroom and/or electronic) and the number of nurses completing each during the past 24 months. Do not include orientation activities or in-service education. Include programs covering each of the following topics: (SE5)
    * Research, including protection of human subjects
    * Evidence-based practice
    * Application of ethical principles
    * *ANA's Bill of Rights for Nurses* (American Nurses Association, 2001a)
    * Professional standards of practice and performance
    * Cultural competence
    * Data and information analysis competencies
    * Quality improvement
    * Leadership

- Nurse Practice Act (or similar document for international applicants)
- Patient privacy, security, and confidentiality
- Regulatory requirements

Exemplary Professional Practice

11. Describe the Professional Practice Model(s) and the Care Delivery System(s) in use in the organization. The *Professional Practice Model* is a schematic description of a theory, phenomenon, or system that depicts how nurses practice, collaborate, communicate, and develop professionally. A *Care Delivery System* delineates nurses' authority and accountability for clinical decision-making and outcomes. If possible, provide a depiction of each model. (EP1, EP1EO, EP2, EP3, EP4, EP5, EP6, EP7, & EP12)

12. Unit-based, nationally benchmarked nurse satisfaction or engagement data for a 2- or 3-year period to include data from the most recent two (2) survey cycles. If available, include the levels of statistical significance as compared to the benchmark. Include a graphic display of the data that clearly identifies benchmarks. (EP3)

13. For U.S. applicants, case mix index information, by unit, service line or product line, for each of the two (2) 1-year periods immediately preceding the submission of written documentation. If this is not feasible, explain why. (EP8)

14. The actual to budgeted direct Nursing Care Hours/Patient Day (HPPD) or hours per workload index by unit for each of the two (2) 1-year periods immediately preceding the submission of written documentation. (EP11)

15. A table of the interdisciplinary committees and task forces at the organizational level, a description of each one's purpose, and guidelines for decision-making. Include nurse membership and role on the committee. Indicate each nurse's work unit(s) and role(s) in the organization. (EP13, EP14, & EP16)

16. Access to the state's Nurse Practice Act. It is sufficient to provide the web address of this document after validating that the most current version of the act is available on the web site. If this is not the case, provide a hard copy of the most current version of the act. (EP19)

17. Performance appraisal tools, if used, and all associated peer evaluation tools for staff nurses and nurse leaders. Include frequency of evaluation. If the organization uses multiple versions of these tools, provide a representative sample for all levels of nurses. (EP20)

18. A description of the process by which the CNO or his or her designeé participates in credentialing, privileging, and evaluating advanced-practice nurses. Include the frequency of re-privileging.

19. The policies and procedures that address patient ethical issues/needs. Describe the leadership of nurses in developing and participating in these programs. (EP23)

20. The policies and procedures that permit and encourage nurses to confidentially express their concerns about their professional practice environment without retribution. (EP28)

21. The policies and procedures that address the identification and management of problems related to incompetent, unsafe, or unprofessional practice or conduct. (EP28)

22. The policies and procedures regarding interdisciplinary conflict. (EP29)

23. Nursing-sensitive indicator data related to patient outcomes for a 2-year period. If available, include the levels of statistical significance as compared to the benchmark. Data at the unit level by measure must be submitted on patient falls, nosocomial pressure ulcer incidence and/or prevalence, along with two (2) (the same data sets as used in response to EP32EO) of the following:
    - Blood stream infections
    - Urinary tract infections
    - Ventilator-associated pneumonia
    - Restraint use
    - Pediatric IV infiltrations
    - Other specialty-specific nationally benchmarked indicators

Include a graphic display of the data that clearly identifies benchmarks. List all external databases used to benchmark your performance. (EP32) Note: By 2012, organizations must provide unit-level data on all applicable indicators listed above.

24. Nursing-sensitive indicator data related to nurse work-related injuries such as needle sticks, musculoskeletal injuries, and exposures (e.g., laser, chemicals, toxins, infectious agents). (EP5, EP15, & EP30)

25. A description of the infrastructure, the organizational committees, and decision-making bodies specifically designed to oversee the quality of patient care. (EP33)

26. Patient satisfaction data at the unit level by measure for a 2-year period, including statistical levels of significance. Include a graphic display of the data that clearly identifies benchmarks. (EP35)

New Knowledge, Innovations, and Improvements
27. The institution's policies, procedures (including Institutional Review Board), and processes that protect the rights of participants in research. (NK2)

28. The credentials or related experience of all external experts and other resources used to develop and/or improve the infrastructures, capacities, and processes for evidence-based practice and research. (NK4 & NK4EO)

COMPONENTS AND SOURCES OF EVIDENCE

This section describes the expectations for each of the five (5) model components and lists the Magnet program requirements as Sources of Evidence. Table 2 depicts the labeling convention used to refer to the Sources of Evidence by Magnet Model component (e.g., TL4 or TL4EO). The Sources of Evidence are further subcategorized for easy understanding (e.g., *Strategic Planning, Advocacy and Influence*, and *Visibility and Accessibility*).

TABLE 2. REFERENCE LABELS OF THE SOURCES OF EVIDENCE

LABEL	MODEL COMPONENT	SOURCE NUMBER	OUTCOME IDENTIFIER
TL	Transformational Leadership	TL1, TL2, etc.	TL3EO, etc
SE	Structural Empowerment	SE1, SE2, etc.	SE2EO, etc.
EP	Exemplary Professional Practice	EP1, EP2, etc.	EP1EO, etc.
NK	New Knowledge, Innovations, and Improvements	NK1, NK2, etc.	NK4EO, etc.
EO	Empirical Outcomes		

Note that the Empirical Outcome (EO) sources are embedded as part of the other four (4) Model components. Writing guidelines for empirical outcomes are described in the Magnet Recognition Program Application Manual chapters 4 (page 34) and 5 (page 52).

For new applicants, Transformational Leadership, Structural Empowerment, and Exemplary Professional Practice will bear heavier weight (highlighted in gold) than New Knowledge, Innovations, and Improvements and Empirical Outcomes. For redesignating organizations, New Knowledge, Innovations, and Improvements and Empirical Outcomes will be more heavily weighted than Transformational Leadership, Structural Empowerment, and Exemplary Professional Practice (see Table 3).

TABLE 3. WEIGHT OF THE COMPONENTS OF THE MAGNET MODEL

NEW APPLICANTS	REDESIGNATING MAGNETS
Transformational Leadership	Transformational Leadership
Structural Empowerment	Structural Empowerment
Exemplary Professional Practice	Exemplary Professional Practice
New Knowledge, Innovations, and Improvements	New Knowledge, Innovations, and Improvements
Empirical Outcomes	Empirical Outcomes

Key: Gold highlights represent more heavily-weighted components

Model Components and Sources of Evidence

This chapter describes the expectations for each of the five model components and the related Sources of Evidence in each component. The Empirical Outcome (EO) sources are embedded in each of the other components: Transformational Leadership, Structural Empowerment, Exemplary Professional Practice and New Knowledge, Innovations & Improvements.

COMPONENTS AND SOURCES OF EVIDENCE

FORCES OF MAGNETISM
- QUALITY OF NURSING LEADERSHIP
- MANAGEMENT STYLE

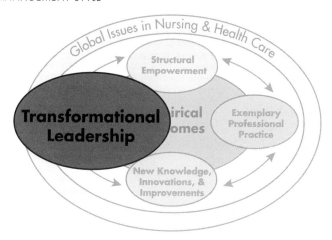

I. Transformational Leadership (TL)

The CNO in a Magnet organization is a knowledgeable, transformational leader who develops a strong vision and well-articulated philosophy, Professional Practice Model, and strategic and quality plans in leading nursing services. The transformational CNO communicates expectations, develops leaders, and evolves the organization to meet current and anticipated needs and strategic priorities. Nursing leaders at all levels of the organization convey a strong sense of advocacy and support on behalf of staff and patients.

The CNO must be strategically positioned within the organization to effectively influence other executive stakeholders, including the board of directors/trustees. Strategic positioning is imperative to achieving the level of influence required to lead others both operationally and during periods of change management due to internal or external factors. Executive-level nursing leaders serve at the top level of the organization, with the CNO typically reporting to the chief executive officer.

The nursing organization must be continually assessed, and appropriate strategic and quality plans for nursing and patient care developed that are congruent with those of the organization. The CNO must secure adequate resources to implement these plans and engage in interdisciplinary efforts to accomplish this work.

Wherever nursing is practiced, the CNO must develop structures, processes, and expectations for staff nurse input and involvement throughout the organization. Mechanisms must be implemented for evidence-based practice to evolve and for innovation to flourish. The CNO should be seen as an executive leader and a nursing advocate and perceived as leading nursing practice and patient care. The CNO is visible, accessible, and communicates effectively in an environment of mutual respect. As a result, nurses throughout the organization should perceive that their voices are heard, their input valued, and their practice supported.

Sources of Evidence

Strategic Planning. Describe and demonstrate

TL1   How nursing's mission, vision, values, and strategic and quality plans reflect the organization's current and anticipated strategic priorities.

TL2   How nurses at every level—CNO, nurse administrators, and direct-care nurses—advocate for resources, including fiscal and technology resources, to support unit/division goals.

TL3   The strategic planning structure(s) and process(es) used by nursing to improve the healthcare system's:
- Effectiveness and
- Efficiency.

TL3EO   The outcome(s) that resulted from the planning described in TL3.

Advocacy and Influence. Describe and demonstrate

TL4   The process(es) that enable the CNO to influence organization-wide changes.

TL4EO   One CNO-influenced organization-wide change.

TL5   How nurse leaders guide the transition during periods of planned or unplanned change.

TL6   How the organization supports:
- Leadership development
- Performance management
- Mentoring activities
- Succession planning for nurse leaders

TL7   How nurse leaders value, encourage, recognize/reward, and implement innovation.

Visibility, Accessibility, and Communication. Describe and demonstrate

TL8   The various methods by which the CNO is visible and accesses direct-care nurses.

TL9   The various methods by which direct-care nurses access nurse leaders.

TL10   How nurse leaders use input from direct-care nurses to improve the work environment and patient care.

TL10EO Changes in the work environment and patient care based on input from the direct-care nurses.

FORCES OF MAGNETISM
- ORGANIZATIONAL STRUCTURE
- PERSONNEL POLICIES AND PROGRAMS
- COMMUNITY AND THE HEALTHCARE ORGANIZATION
- IMAGE OF NURSING
- PROFESSIONAL DEVELOPMENT

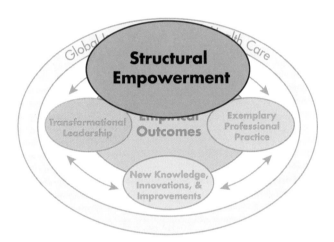

II. Structural Empowerment (SE)

Magnet structural environments are generally flat, flexible, and decentralized. Nurses throughout the organization are involved in self-governance and decision-making structures and processes that establish standards of practice and address issues of concern. The flow of information and decision-making is bi-directional and horizontal between and among professional nurses at the bedside, the leadership team, and the CNO. The CNO serves on the highest-level councils and/ or committees. Nurse leaders throughout the organization also serve on committees and task forces that address excellence in patient care and the safe, efficient, and effective operation of the organization.

The healthcare organization promotes relationships among all types of community organizations to develop strong partnerships to improve patient outcomes and the health of the communities they serve. Magnet nurses extend their influence to professional and community groups, advancing the nursing profession and supporting organizational goals, and personal and professional growth and development.

The organization uses multiple strategies to establish structures, systematic and equitable processes, and expectations that support lifelong professional learning, role development, and career advancement. Relationships are established throughout the organization and with the community to encourage educational advancement.

Nurse contributions to the organization and community are recognized for their positive effect on patients and families. Nurses are acknowledged in various and substantive ways for these accomplishments, enhancing the image of nursing in the community.

Sources of Evidence

Professional Engagement. Describe and demonstrate

SE1 The structure(s) and process(es) that enable nurses from all settings and roles to actively participate in organizational decision-making groups such as committees, councils, and task forces.

SE1EO Two improvements in different practice settings because of nurse involvement in organizational decision-making groups such as committees, councils, and task forces.

SE2 The structure(s) and process(es) that enable nurses at all levels to participate in professional nursing organizations at the local, state, and national levels. Include international participation, if any.

SE2EO Two improvements in different practice settings that occurred because of nurse involvement in a professional nursing organization(s).

Commitment to Professional Development. Describe and demonstrate

SE3 How the organization sets expectations and supports nurses at all levels who seek additional formal nursing education (e.g., baccalaureate, master's, doctoral degrees).

SE3EO That the organization has met goals for improvement in formal education. Graphically summarize at least 2 years of data to display changes over time.

SE4 How the organization sets goals and supports professional development and professional certification, such as tuition/registration reimbursement and participation in external local, regional, national, and international conferences or meetings.

SE4EO   That the organization has met goals for improvement in professional certification. Graphically summarize at least 2 years of data to display changes over time. Include participation of nurses in all specialties.

SE5   The structure(s) and process(es) used by nursing to develop and provide continuing education programs for nurses at all levels and settings. Include how the organization provides onsite internal electronic and classroom methods. Do not include orientation.

SE5EO   The effectiveness of two educational programs provided in SE5.

SE6   How the organization provides career development opportunities for non-nurse employees and members of the community interested in becoming nurses.

Teaching and Role Development. Describe and demonstrate

SE7   The structure(s) and process(es) used by the organization to promote the teaching role of nurses. Include examples related to patients and staff members.

SE8   How nursing facilitates the effective transition of new graduate nurses into the work environment.

SE9   How nurses support community educational activities.

SE10   How nurses support academic practicum experiences and serve as preceptors, instructors, adjunct faculty, or faculty.

Commitment to Community Involvement. Describe and demonstrate

SE11   The structure(s) and process(es) used to identify and allocate resources for affiliations with schools of nursing, consortiums, or community outreach programs.

SE11EO   The result(s) of the affiliations with schools of nursing, consortiums, or community outreach programs described in SE11.

SE12   How the organization supports and recognizes the participation of nurses at all levels in service to the community.

SE13   How the organization or nursing addresses the healthcare needs of the community by establishing partnerships.

Recognition of Nursing. Describe and demonstrate

SE14   The structure(s) and process(es) the organization uses to recognize and make visible the contributions of nurses.

SE15   That the nursing community and the community at large (e.g., local, state, national, international) recognize the value of nursing in the organization.

FORCES OF MAGNETISM
- PROFESSIONAL MODELS OF CARE
- CONSULTATION AND RESOURCES
- AUTONOMY
- NURSES AS TEACHERS
- INTERDISCIPLINARY RELATIONSHIPS
- QUALITY OF CARE: ETHICS, PATIENT SAFETY AND QUALITY INFRASTRUCTURE
- QUALITY IMPROVEMENT

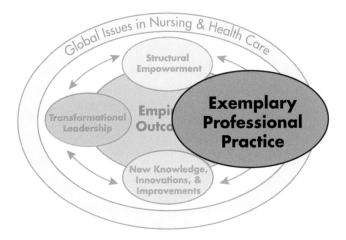

III. Exemplary Professional Practice (EP)

A Professional Practice Model is the overarching conceptual framework for nurses, nursing care, and interdisciplinary patient care. It is a schematic description of a system, theory, or phenomenon that depicts how nurses practice, collaborate, communicate, and develop professionally to provide the highest quality care for those served by the organization (e.g., patients, families, community). The Professional Practice Model illustrates the alignment and integration of nursing practice with the mission, vision, philosophy, and values that nursing has adapted. Magnet hospitals take the lead in research efforts to create and test models of professional practice for nurses.

The Care Delivery System is integrated within the Professional Practice Model and promotes continuous, consistent, efficient, and accountable delivery of nursing care. The Care Delivery System is adapted to regulatory considerations and describes the manner in which care is delivered, skill set required, context of care, and expected outcomes of care. Nurses create patient care delivery systems that delineate the nurses' authority and accountability for clinical decision-making and outcomes. At the organizational level, nurse leaders ensure that care is patient/family centered.

Exemplary professional practice is evident in Magnet hospitals. Nurses have significant control over staffing and scheduling processes and work in collaboration with interdisciplinary partners to achieve high-quality patient outcomes.

Interdisciplinary collaboration is evident with clear expectations and direction to all practicing nurses about the importance of partnerships with patients and families, and with the disciplines of medicine, pharmacy, nutrition, rehabilitation, social work, psychology, and other professions to ensure a comprehensive care plan. Collegial working relationships within and among the disciplines are valued by the organization and its employees. Mutual respect is based on the premise that all members of the healthcare team make essential and meaningful contributions in the achievement of clinical outcomes. Conflict management strategies are in place and used effectively, when indicated.

The autonomous nurse makes judgments about how to provide care based on the unique needs and attributes of the patient and family. The knowledge, skills, and resources that have been identified by the nursing staff as necessary to practice are consistently available in the practice environment. These resources form the basis of the Care Delivery System. Competency assessment and peer evaluation ensures that the nurse bases care delivery decisions on current evidence about safe and ethical practice using the nursing process.

Attention is given to achieving equity in care. Workplace advocacy initiatives address ethical issues and the privacy, security, and confidentiality of patients and staff.

The achievement of exemplary professional practice is grounded by a culture of safety, quality monitoring, and quality improvement. Nurses collaborate with other disciplines to ensure that care is comprehensive, coordinated, and monitored for effectiveness through the quality improvement model. Nurses participate in safety initiatives that incorporate national best practices. Sufficient resources are available to respond to safety initiatives and quality improvements for patients and employees.

Nurses at all levels analyze data and use national benchmarks to gain a comparative perspective about their performance and the care patients receive. Action plans are developed that lead to systematic improvements over time. Magnet hospital data demonstrate outcome measures that outperform the benchmark statistic of the national database used in patient and nursing-sensitive indicators the majority of the time.

Sources of Evidence

Professional Practice Model. Describe and demonstrate

EP1   How nurses develop, apply, evaluate, adapt, and modify the Professional Practice Model.

EP1EO The result of applying the Professional Practice Model. Include two examples related to nursing practice, collaboration, communication, or professional development activities.

EP2   How nurses investigate, develop, implement, and systematically evaluate standards of practice and standards of care.

EP3   The structure(s) and process(es) that include direct-care nurse involvement in tracking and analyzing nurse satisfaction or engagement data.

EP3EO That nurse satisfaction or engagement data aggregated at the organization or unit level outperform the mean, median or other benchmark statistic of the national database used. Include participation rates, analysis, and evaluation of the data.

Care Delivery System(s). Describe and demonstrate

EP4   That the structure(s) and process(es) of the Care Delivery System(s) involve the patient and/or his or her support system in the planning and delivery of care. Provide at least two examples of a plan of care that included patient and/or family member involvement.

EP5   How nurses use the Care Delivery System(s) to make patient care assignments that ensure continuity, quality, and effectiveness of care within and across services and settings.

EP6   How regulatory and professional standards are incorporated into the Care Delivery System(s).

EP7   The structure(s) and process(es) used to engage internal experts and external consultants to improve care in the practice setting.

EP7EO   Two improvements in the practice setting that occurred as a result of the use of internal experts or external consultants.

Staffing, Scheduling, and Budgeting Processes. Describe and demonstrate

EP8   How nurses use trended data to formulate the staffing plan and acquire necessary resources to assure consistent application of the Care Delivery System(s).

EP9   How direct-care nurses participate in staffing and scheduling processes.

EP10   How nurses develop, implement, and evaluate action plans related to unit-based staff recruitment and retention.

EP11   How guidelines such as the ANA Principles of Nurse Staffing (American Nurses Association, 2005) standards for scheduling, delegation, and from nursing specialty organizations and/or state-mandated requirements are incorporated into staffing and scheduling processes.

EP12   How nurses analyze data to guide decisions regarding unit and department budget formulation, implementation, monitoring, and evaluation.

Interdisciplinary Care. Describe and demonstrate

EP13   How nurses have assumed leadership roles in interdisciplinary collaboration.

EP14   How the organization ensures the participation of nurses at all levels in interdisciplinary activities to develop policy and standards of care.

EP15   Interdisciplinary collaboration using continuous quality and process improvement.

EP16   Interdisciplinary collaboration across multiple settings to ensure the continuum of care.

EP17   Interdisciplinary collaboration to ensure that information systems and technology used for clinical care monitoring, documentation, and communication are integrated and evaluated.

EP18   Interdisciplinary collaboration to develop, implement, and evaluate a comprehensive set of patient education programs and resources within the organization.

Accountability, Competence, and Autonomy. Describe and demonstrate

EP19   That nurses have ready access to, and routinely use, current literature, professional standards, and other data sources to support autonomous practice.

EP20   That nurses at all levels routinely use self-appraisal performance review and peer review, including annual goal setting, for the assurance of competence and professional development.

EP21   The structure(s) and process(es) that support shared leadership/participative decision-making and promote nursing autonomy.

EP22   That nurses are accountable to resolve issues related to patient care or operational issues.

Ethics, Privacy, Security, and Confidentiality. Describe and demonstrate

EP23   How nurses use available resources, such as the ANA Code of Ethics for Nurses (American Nurses Association, 2001b) to address complex ethical issues. Provide examples from different practice settings.

EP24   How nurses have resolved issues related to patient privacy, security, and confidentiality.

Diversity and Workplace Advocacy. Describe and demonstrate

EP25   How the organization identifies and addresses disparities in the management of the healthcare needs of diverse patient populations. Include the role of the nurse.

EP26   How nurses use resources to meet the unique and individual needs of patients.

EP27   How the organization promotes a non-discriminatory climate for patients.

EP28   The organizational structure(s) and process(es) that are in place to identify and manage problems related to incompetent, unsafe, or unprofessional conduct.

EP29   The organization's workplace advocacy initiatives for:
- Caregiver stress
- Diversity
- Rights
- Confidentiality

Culture of Safety. Describe and demonstrate

EP30   The structure(s) and process(es) used by the organization to improve workplace safety for nurses, based on recommendations such as the ANA's Safe Patient Handling and Movement (**www.nursingworld.org/ MainMenuCategories/ANAPoliticalPower/Federal/Issues/ SPHM.aspx**).

EP30EO   Two workplace safety improvements for nurses that resulted from the structure(s) and process(es) in EP30.

EP31   How the organization uses a facility-wide approach for proactive risk assessment and error management.

EP32   The nursing structure(s) and process(es) that support a culture of patient safety.

EP32EO   That nursing sensitive indicator data aggregated at the organization or unit level outperform the mean, median or other benchmark statistic of the national database used. Provide analysis and evaluation of data related to patient falls, nosocomial pressure ulcer prevalence and/or incidence, and two of the following:
- Blood stream infections
- Urinary tract infections
- Ventilator-associated pneumonia
- Restraint use
- Pediatric IV infiltrations
- Other specialty-specific nationally benchmarked indicators (use only for units for which the above do not apply)

Quality Care Monitoring and Improvement. Describe and demonstrate

EP33   The structure(s) and process(es) used by the organization to allocate and/or reallocate resources to monitor and improve the quality of nursing, and total patient care. The nurse has responsibility for ensuring the coordination of care among other disciplines and support staff.

EP33EO   How the allocation and/or reallocation of resources improved the quality of nursing care.

EP34   How nurse leaders ensure the dissemination of comprehensive quality data to direct-care nurses.

EP35   The structure(s) and process(es) used to identify significant findings and trends in overall patient satisfaction with nursing as compared to benchmarked sources.

EP35EO   That patient satisfaction data aggregated at the organization or unit level outperform the mean, median or other benchmark statistic of the national database used. Provide analysis and evaluation of data and resultant action plans related to patient satisfaction with nursing addressing four of the following:

• Pain

• Education

• Courtesy and respect from nurses

• Careful listening by nurses

• Response time

• Other nurse-related national survey questions

FORCES OF MAGNETISM
- QUALITY OF CARE: RESEARCH AND
  EVIDENCE-BASED PRACTICE
- QUALITY IMPROVEMENT

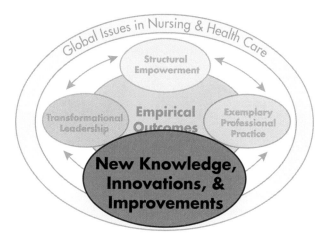

IV. New Knowledge, Innovations, and Improvements (NK)

Magnet organizations conscientiously integrate evidence-based practice and research into clinical and operational processes. Nurses are educated about evidence-based practice and research, enabling them to appropriately explore the safest and best practices for their patients and practice environment, and to generate new knowledge.

Published research is systematically evaluated and used. Nurses serve on the board that reviews proposals for research, and knowledge gained through research is disseminated to the community of nurses.

Organizations achieving Magnet recognition possess established and evolving programs related to evidence-based practices and research programs. Infrastructures and resources are in place to support the advancement of evidence-based practices and research in all clinical settings. Targets for research productivity are set with participation and leadership in a multitude of research activities within the framework of the practice site.

Innovations in patient care, nursing, and the practice environment are the hallmark of organizations receiving Magnet recognition. Establishing new ways of achieving high-quality, effective, and efficient care is the outcome of transformational leadership, empowering structures and processes, and exemplary professional practice in nursing.

Sources of Evidence

Research. Describe and demonstrate

NK1   That nurses at all levels evaluate and use published research findings in their practice.

NK2   Consistent membership and involvement by at least one nurse in the governing body responsible for the protection of human subjects in research, and that a nurse votes on nursing-related protocols.

NK3   That direct-care nurses support the human rights of participants in research.

NK4   The structure(s) and process(es) used by the organization to develop, expand, and/or advance nursing research.

NK4EO   Nursing research studies from the past 2 years, ongoing or completed, generated from the structure(s) and process(es) in NK4. Provide a table including:
  • Study title
  • Study status
  • Principal investigator name(s)
  • Principal investigator credential(s)
  • Role(s) of nurses in the study
  • Study scope (internal to a single organization, multiple organizations within a system, independent organizations collaboratively)
  • Study type (replication—yes or no; qualitative, quantitative, or both)
  Select one completed research study and respond to the four criteria listed in the EO guidelines provided on page 32.

NK5   How the organization disseminates knowledge generated through nursing research to internal and external audiences.

Evidence-Based Practice. Describe and demonstrate

NK6   The structure(s) and process(es) used to evaluate existing nursing practice, based on evidence.

NK7   The structure(s) and process(es) used to translate new knowledge into nursing practice.

NK7EO   How translation of new knowledge into nursing practice has affected patient outcomes.

Innovation. Describe and demonstrate

NK8   Innovations in nursing practice.

NK9   The structure(s) and process(es) by which nurses are involved with the evaluation and allocation of technology and information systems to support practice, or nurses' participation in architecture and space design to support practice.

NK9EO   An improvement in practice due to nurse involvement in technology and information system decision-making, or due to nurses' participation in architecture and space design.

FORCES OF MAGNETISM
• QUALITY CARE

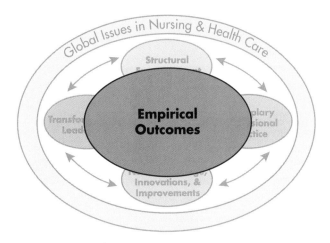

V. Empirical Outcomes (EO)

Nursing makes an essential contribution to patient, nursing workforce, organizational, and consumer outcomes. The empirical measurement of quality outcomes related to nursing leadership and clinical practice in Magnet organizations is imperative. In each of the other model components, the EOs are requested as Sources of Evidence.

Display of data using graphs and charts is an excellent way to illustrate outcomes. When documenting evidence in response to an EO, unless already addressed in the associated Source of Evidence, include the following information in the response:
• Describe the purpose and the background.
• Describe how the work was done (methods or approach).
• Discuss who (CNO, staff RNs, CFO, APRNs, pharmacists, physicians, etc.) was involved and what units participated.
• Describe the measurement used to evaluate the outcomes and the impact (show results and significance of the results).

The relationships among the structure and processes of care and associated outcomes need to be continually assessed and monitored. EOs focus on the results and the differences that can be demonstrated based on the application of sound structure and processes in the healthcare team, organization, and systems of care.

Outcomes are dynamic and define areas of both improved performance and those requiring additional effort to achieve improvement. Organizations must establish baselines for measures and track progress over time compared to the baseline and national benchmarks. Magnet organizations are expected to serve as mentors and lead the way in the provision of quality patient care and the creation of environments that contribute to the well-being of the workforce and the community at large.

References

American Hospital Association. (2007). *Fast facts on US hospitals* [last updated October 23, 2007]. Last accessed April 7, 2000, from http://www.aha.org/ aha/resource-center/Statistics-and-Studies/fast-facts.html.

American Nurses Association. (1979). *The study of credentialing in nursing: A new approach* (Vol. I, Report of the Committee). Kansas City, MO: Author.

American Nurses Association. (2000). *Scope and standards of practice for nursing professional development*. Washington, DC: Author.

American Nurses Association. (2001a). *ANA's bill of rights for registered nurses*. Washington, DC: Author.

American Nurses Association. (2001b). *Code of ethics for nurses, with interpretive statements*. Washington, DC: Author.

American Nurses Association. (2004). *Scope and standards for nurse administrators* (2nd ed.). Washington, DC: Author.

American Nurses Association. (2005). *Principles for nurse staffing* (Appendix A). In *Utilization guide for the ANA principles for nurse staffing* (pp. 20–28). Silver Spring, MD: Author.

American Nurses Credentialing Center. (2004). *Magnet Recognition Program: Application Manual 2005*. Silver Spring, MD: Author.

Burns, J. (1978). *Leadership*. New York: Harper & Row.

Burns, N., & Grove, S. K. (2005). *The practice of nursing research: Conduct, critique, and utilization* (5th ed.). St. Louis, MO: Elsevier.

Centers for Medicare and Medicaid Services. (2006, June). *Revised long-term-care facility resident assessment instrument user's manual* (Version 2.0, rev.). Washington, DC: U.S. Department of Health and Human Services, Author.

Corley, M. C., Minick, P., Elswick, R. K., & Jacobs, M. (2005). Nurse moral distress and ethical work environment. *Nursing Ethics*, 12(4), 382–390.

Donabedian, A. (1980). *The definition of quality and approaches to its assessment*. Ann Arbor, MI: Health Administration Press.

Donabedian, A. (2003). *An introduction to quality assurance in health care*. New York: Oxford University Press.

Dunham-Taylor, J. (2000). Nurse executive transformational leadership found in participative organizations. *Journal of Nursing Administration*, 30(5), 241–250.

Farquharson, J.M. (2004). Liability of the nurse manager. In T.D. Aiken (Ed.), *Legal, ethical, and political issues in nursing* (2nd ed.) (pp. 311-336). Philadelphia, PA: F.A. Davis Company.

Greenhalgh, T. (2004). Diffusion of innovations in service organizations: Systematic review and recommendations. *The Milbank Quarterly*, 82, 581–6.

Griffith, J. R., & White, K. R. (2002). *The well-managed healthcare organization* (5th ed.). Chicago: Health Administration Press.

Hinshaw, A.S. (2002). Building magnetism into health organizations. In M.L. McClure & A.S. Hinshaw (Eds.), *Magnet hospitals revisited: Attraction and retention of professional nurses* (pp. 83-102). Washington, DC: American Nurses Association.

Institute of Medicine. (2003). *Health professions education: A bridge to quality.* Washington, DC: National Academy Press.

Lynn, J., Baily, M. A., Bottrell, M., et al. (2007). The ethics of using quality improvement methods in health care. *Annals of Internal Medicine*, 146, 666–673.

MacDonald, C. (2002). Nurse autonomy as relational. *Nursing Ethics*, 9, 194-201.

National Quality Forum. (2004). *National voluntary consensus standards for nursing home care.* Washington, DC: Author.

Needleman, J., Buerhaus, P., Mattke, S., Stewart, M., & Zelevinsky, K. (2002). Nurse-staffing levels and the quality of care in hospitals. *New England Journal of Medicine*, 346(22), 1715–1722.

Polit, D., & Hungler, B. (1995). *Nursing research: Principles and methods.* Philadelphia: Lippincott.

Sackett, D. L., Straus, S. E., Richardson, W. S., Rosenberg, W., & Haynes, R. B. (2000). *Evidence based medicine: How to practice and teach EBM* (2nd ed.). Edinburgh: Churchill Livingstone.

Schaufeli, W., Salanova, M., González-romá, V., & Bakker, A. (2002). The measurement of engagement and burnout: A two sample confirmatory factor analytic approach. *Journal of Happiness Studies*, 3(1), 71–92.

Scott, J., & Marshall, G. (Eds.). (2005). *A dictionary of sociology.* New York: Oxford University Press.

Tranmer, J. (2005). Autonomy and decision-making in nursing. In L. McGillis Hall (Ed.), *Quality work environments for nurse and patient safety* (pp. 139-162). Sudbury, MA: Jones and Bartlett Publishers.

Urden, L. D., & Monarch, K. (2002). The ANCC Magnet Recognition Program: Converting research findings into action. In M. L. McClure & A. S. Hinshaw (Eds.), *Magnet hospitals revisited: Attraction and retention of professional nurses* (pp. 103–116). Washington, DC: American Nurses Association.

U.S. Department of Health and Human Services. (n.d.). Code of Federal Regulations Title 45 Public Welfare Part 46: Protection of Human Subjects, Title 21 Food and Drugs Part 50: Protection of Human Subjects. Washington, DC: Author.

Wade, G. (1999). Professional nurse autonomy: Concept analysis and application to nursing education. *Journal of Advanced Nursing*, 30, 301-318.

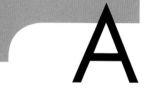

Forces of Magnetism

1. **Quality of nursing leadership**—Nursing leaders were perceived as knowledgeable, strong risk-takers who followed an articulated philosophy in the day-to-day operations of the nursing department. Nursing leaders also conveyed a strong sense of advocacy and support on behalf of the staff.

   Expectations of a Magnet Organization 2005: Knowledgeable, strong, risk-taking nurse leaders follow a well-articulated, strategic, and visionary philosophy in the day-to-day operations of the nursing services. Nursing leaders, at all levels of the organization, convey a strong sense of advocacy and support for the staff and for the patient. (The results of quality leadership are evident in nursing practice at the patient's side.)

2. **Organizational structure**—Organizational structures were characterized as flat, rather than tall, and where unit-based decision-making prevailed. Nursing departments were decentralized, with strong nursing representation evident in the organizational committee structure. The nursing leader served at the executive level of the organization, and the chief nursing officer (CNO) reported to the chief executive officer.

   Expectations of a Magnet Organization 2005: Organizational structures are generally flat, rather than tall, and decentralized decision-making prevails. The organizational structure is dynamic and responsive to change. Strong nursing representation is evident in the organizational committee structure. Executive-level nursing leaders serve at the executive level of the organization. The CNO typically reports directly to the chief executive officer. The organization has a functioning and productive system of shared decision-making.

3. **Management style**—Hospital and nursing administrators were found to use a participative management style, incorporating feedback from staff at all levels of the organization. Feedback was characterized as encouraged and valued. Nurses serving in leadership positions were visible, accessible, and committed to communicating effectively with staff.

   Expectations of a Magnet Organization 2005: Healthcare organization and nursing leaders create an environment supporting participation. Feedback is encouraged and valued and is incorporated from the staff at all levels of the organization. Nurses serving in leadership positions are visible, accessible, and committed to communicating effectively with staff.

4. **Personnel policies and programs**—Salaries and benefits were characterized as competitive. Rotating shifts were minimized, and creative and flexible staffing models were used. Personnel policies were created with staff involvement, and significant administrative and clinical promotional opportunities existed.

   Expectations of a Magnet Organization 2005: Salaries and benefits are competitive. Creative and flexible staffing models that support a safe and healthy work environment are used. Personnel policies are created with direct-care nurse involvement. Significant opportunities for professional growth exist in administrative and clinical tracks. Personnel policies and programs support professional nursing practice, work/life balance, and the delivery of quality care.

5. **Professional models of care**—Models of care were used that gave nurses the responsibility and authority for the provision of patient care. Nurses were accountable for their own practice and were the coordinators of care.

   Expectations of a Magnet Organization 2005: There are models of care that give nurses the responsibility and authority for the provision of direct patient care. Nurses are accountable for their own practice as well as the coordination of care. The models of care (i.e., primary nursing, case management, family-centered, district, and holistic) provide for the continuity of care across the continuum. The models take into consideration patients' unique needs and provide skilled nurses and adequate resources to accomplish desired outcomes.

6. **Quality of care**—Nurses perceived that they were providing high-quality care to their patients. Providing quality care was seen as an organizational priority as well, and nurses serving in leadership positions were viewed as responsible for developing the environment in which high quality care could be provided.

   Expectations of a Magnet Organization 2005: Quality is the systematic driving force for nursing and the organization. Nurses serving in leadership positions are responsible for providing an environment that positively influences patient outcomes. There is a pervasive perception among nurses that they provide high-quality care to patients/residents/clients.

7. **Quality improvement**—Quality improvement activities were viewed as educational. Staff nurses participated in the quality improvement process and perceived the process as one that improved the quality of care delivered within the organization.

   Expectations of a Magnet Organization 2005: The organization has structures and processes for the measurement of quality and programs for improving the quality of care and services within the organization.

8. **Consultation and resources**—Adequate consultation and other human resources were available. Knowledgeable experts, particularly advanced-practice nurses, were available and used. In addition, peer support was given within and outside the nursing division.

   Expectations of a Magnet Organization 2005: The healthcare organization provides adequate resources, support, and opportunities for the utilization of experts, particularly advanced-practice nurses. In addition, the organization promotes involvement of nurses in professional organizations and among peers in the community.

9. **Autonomy**—Nurses were permitted and expected to practice autonomously, consistent with professional standards. Independent judgment was expected to be exercised within the context of a multidisciplinary approach to patient care.

   Expectations of a Magnet Organization 2005: Autonomous nursing care is the ability of a nurse to assess and provide nursing actions as appropriate for patient care based on competence, professional expertise, and knowledge. The nurse is expected to practice autonomously, consistent with professional standards. Independent judgment is expected to be exercised within the context of interdisciplinary and multidisciplinary approaches to patient/resident/client care.

10. **Community and the hospital**—Hospitals that were best able to recruit and retain nurses also maintained a strong community presence. A community presence was seen in a variety of ongoing, long-term outreach programs. These outreach programs resulted in the hospital being perceived as a strong, positive, and productive corporate citizen.

    Expectations of a Magnet Organization 2005: Relationships are established within and among all types of healthcare organizations and other community organizations, to develop strong partnerships that support improved client outcomes and the health of the communities they serve.

11. **Nurses as teachers**—Nurses were permitted and expected to incorporate teaching in all aspects of their practice. Teaching was one activity that reportedly gave nurses a great deal of professional satisfaction.

    Expectations of a Magnet Organization 2005: Professional nurses are involved in educational activities within the organization and community. Students from a variety of academic programs are welcomed and supported in the organization; contractual arrangements are mutually beneficial. There is a development and mentoring program for staff preceptors for all levels of students (e.g., students, new graduates, experienced nurses). Staff in all positions serve as faculty and preceptors for students from a variety of academic programs. There is a patient education program that meets the diverse needs of patients in all of the care settings of the organization.

12. **Image of nursing**—Nurses were viewed as integral to the hospital's ability to provide patient care services. The services provided by nurses were characterized as essential to other members of the healthcare team.

    Expectations of a Magnet Organization 2005: The services provided by nurses are characterized as essential by other members of the healthcare team. Nurses are viewed as integral to the healthcare organization's ability to provide patient care. Nurses effectively influence system-wide processes.

13. **Interdisciplinary relationships**—Interdisciplinary relationships were characterized as positive. A sense of mutual respect was exhibited among all disciplines.

    Expectations of a Magnet Organization 2005: Collaborative working relationships within and among the disciplines are valued. Mutual respect is based on the premise that all members of the healthcare team make essential and meaningful contributions in the achievement of clinical outcomes. Conflict management strategies are in place and are used effectively, when indicated.

14. **Professional development**—Significant emphasis was placed on orientation, in-service education, continuing education, formal education, and career development. Personal and professional growth and development were valued. In addition, opportunities for competency-based clinical advancement existed, along with the resources to maintain competency.

    Expectations of a Magnet Organization 2005: The healthcare organization values and supports the personal and professional growth and development of staff. In addition to quality orientation and in-service education addressed earlier in Force 11, emphasis is placed on providing career development services. Programs that promote formal education, professional certification, and career development are evident. Competency-based clinical and leadership/management development is promoted, and adequate human and fiscal resources for all professional development programs are provided.

Sources: American Nurses Credentialing Center (2004, pp. 36–65), Urden and Monarch (2002, pp. 106–107).

Magnet Dictionary

accountability. The ethical concept of being answerable or responsible for one's actions. In nursing, personal accountability is the responsibility nurses have to themselves and to patients and public accountability is the responsibility nurses have to their employers and to society in general. "The primary goals of professional accountability in nursing are to maintain high standards of care and to protect the patient from harm. All nurses are accountable for the proper use of their knowledge and skills in the provision of care" (Farquharson, 2004, p. 311-312).

acute care. A healthcare organization in which care is delivered to hospitalized patients.

advanced-practice nurse (APRN). A registered nurse who has met advanced educational and clinical practice requirements beyond the 2–4 years of basic nursing education required of all RNs. Under this umbrella are four principal types of APRNs: nurse practitioners, certified nurse midwives, clinical nurse specialists, and certified registered nurse anesthetists.

all level of nurses. See *nurses at every level.*

ambulatory clinic. A facility in which people typically other than inpatients visit providers for treatment and/or health counseling.

autonomy. "Professional nurse autonomy implies the right to exercise clinical and organizational judgment within the context of an interdependent health care team and in accordance with the socially and legally granted freedom of the discipline" (MacDonald, 2002, as cited in Tranmer, 2005, p. 141). "Organizational autonomy is an environmental characteristic that involves nurses in the broader unit and hospital decision-making processes pertaining to patient care. Clinical autonomy and organizational autonomy or control over nursing practice are interactive concepts" (Hinshaw, 2002, p. 92-93).

beds. Operating beds for the care of patients staying 24 hours or more (category does not include bassinets).

benchmarking. Comparing data from the organization and other sources for the purpose of goal setting and performance measurements. To incorporate best practices into an organization's goal setting and performance measurement, benchmarking must use external as well as internal reference points. The contribution of data to benchmarking processes is an essential element of both research and quality improvement efforts in a variety of industries.

care delivery system. A system for the provision of care that delineates the nurses' authority and accountability for clinical decision-making and outcomes. The care delivery system is integrated with the practice model and promotes continuous, consistent, efficient, and accountable nursing care. The care delivery system is adapted to regulatory considerations and describes the context of care, the manner in which care is delivered, skill set required, and expected outcomes of care.

caregiver stress. Also called *moral distress*, a response experience when a decision-maker's ability to carry out a chosen ethical or moral action is thwarted by an individual, institutional, or societal constraint (Corley, Minick, Elswick, and Jacobs, 2005).

case mix index. A numerical score used in the United States as a descriptor at the organization level of the relative resource use for the *average* patient/client/resident. This use is computed using data on the characteristics and clinical needs of the patients/clients/residents served by the organization.

certification. A process by which a nongovernmental agency or association certifies that an individual licensed to practice a profession has met certain predetermined standards specified by that profession for specialty practice. Its purpose is to ensure various publics that an individual has mastered a body of knowledge and acquired skills in a particular specialty (American Nurses Association, 1979, p. 67). Certifications for ability to perform clinical interventions (e.g., Advanced Cardiac Life Support [ACLS], Basic Life Support [BLS], Neonatal Resuscitation Program [NRP], Pediatric Advanced Life Support [PALS]) are not included.

chief nursing officer (CNO). The nurse who participates in the management of healthcare services delivery by directing and coordinating the work of nursing and other personnel and representing nursing services.

competence. The Institute of Medicine (2003) defined *professional competence* as "the habitual and judicious use of communication, knowledge, technical skills, clinical reasoning, emotions, values, and reflection in daily practice for the benefit of the individuals and community being served" (p. 24).

complaint. A written statement expressing dissatisfaction with, for example, service, practice, or professionalism. In contrast, a grievance is a formal complaint filed for resolution with a grievance system or process.

continuing education. Systematic professional learning experiences designed to augment the knowledge, skills, and attitudes of nurses' contributions to quality health care and their pursuit of professional career goals.

direct-care nurse. The nurse providing care directly to patients, excluding the nurse manager and nurse executive. (However, in some settings, the nurse manager does spend a portion of her or his work hours providing direct patient care.) Direct-care activities can be reflected as partial full-time equivalents (FTEs).

domain. A meaningful set of related concepts or indicators.

enculturation. A term synonymous with *socialization*, emphasizing that individuals have to constantly learn and use, both formally and informally, the prescribed patterns of cultural behavior in order to become full members of a culture or subculture. It is distinct from *acculturation*, which is synonymous with *assimilation*, a process by which an outsider/group becomes indistinguishably integrated into the dominant society (Scott and Marshall, 2005).

entity. A stand-alone group, whether or not within a system, whose nursing is governed by a CNO or a designated RN executive leader as identified in this glossary and whether or not separately legally established as a for-profit or non-profit, corporation, association, sole proprietorship, or partnership.

evidence-based practice (EBP). The conscientious use/integration of the best research evidence with clinical expertise and patient preferences in nursing practice (adapted from Sackett et al., 2000). EBP is a science-to-service model of engagement of critical thinking to apply research-based evidence (scientific knowledge) and practice-based evidence (art of nursing) within the context of patient values to deliver quality, cost-sensitive care. It is distinguished from *practice-based evidence (PBE)*, a practice-to-science model in which data are derived from interventions thought to be effective but for which empirical evidence is lacking. Providers are engaged in data collection, analysis, and synthesis to inform practice.

hospital system. The American Hospital Association (2007) defines *system* as "either a multihospital or a diversified single hospital system. A *multihospital system* is two or more hospitals owned, leased, sponsored, or contract managed by a central organization. *Single, freestanding* hospitals may be categorized as a system by bringing into membership three or more, and at least 25%, of their owned or leased non-hospital preacute or postacute healthcare organizations. System affiliation does not preclude network participation" (emphasis added).

hours per patient day (HPPD). Nursing care hours; direct hours of nursing care that are *patient* related, including nursing activities that occur away from the patient (e.g., care coordination, documentation time, treatment planning). This category does *not* include indirect hours, nonproductive time, or all-paid hours (e.g., vacation, sick time, orientation, education leave) and does *not* include committee time if the staff person is replaced by another direct caregiver. HPPD is calculated by the total number of direct RN nursing care hours divided by the patient/resident/client census for the same period.

innovation. "*Innovation* in service delivery and organization [is] a novel set of behaviors, routines, and ways of working that are directed at improving health outcomes, administrative efficiency, cost effectiveness, or users' experience and that are implemented by planned and coordinated actions" (Greenhalgh, 2004, emphasis added).

in-service education. Learning experiences provided in the work setting for the purpose of assisting staff members in performing their assigned functions in that particular agency or institution (American Nurses Association, 2000, p. 24).

Institutional Review Board (IRB). An independent committee comprised of scientific, non-scientific, and non-affiliated members established according to the requirements of U.S. federal regulations. Any board, committee, or other group formally designated by an organization to review research involving humans as participants, to approve the initiation of and conduct periodic review of such research. The term includes, but is not limited to, Institutional Review Boards, Investigational Review Boards, Central Review Boards, Independent Review Boards, and Cooperative Research Boards (U.S. Department of Health and Human Services, n.d., [45 CFR §46.402(g)] [21 CFR §50.3(i)]).

interdisciplinary. Reliant on the overlapping skills and knowledge of each team member and discipline, resulting in synergistic effects in which outcomes are improved and more comprehensive than the simple aggregation of any team member's individual efforts.

licensure/registration. The process of granting permission to engage in a specified activity or to perform a specified act. Permission generally is granted following confirmation of knowledge and abilities as evidenced by written, verbal, and/or demonstrated competencies in the performance or engagement of the specified activity or activities.

long-term care. A healthcare organization in which elderly and frail individuals reside.

multidisciplinary. Reliant on each team member or discipline contributing discipline-specific skills.

national certification. See *certification.*

National Labor Relations Board (NLRB). In the United States, the organization established to mediate and adjudicate collective-bargaining disputes regarding employment issues. See www.nlrb.gov.

new graduate. A nurse in first employment following completion of registered nurse education in the United States.

nurse. Generically, the registered professional nurse.

nurse administrator. A registered nurse whose primary responsibility is the management of healthcare services delivery and who represents nursing. For the purposes of this document, the two levels of nurse administrators are those of the *nurse executive* and the *nurse manager* (see entries below).

nurse engagement. A positive emotional connection to a nurses's work. Engagement as defined by Schaufeli, Salanova, González-romá, and Bakker (2002) is characterized by three dimensions: vigor, dedication, and absorption.

nurse leader. A nurse who participates in decision-making bodies and/or has a leadership role.

nurse manager. The nurse who manages one or more defined areas within organized nursing services. His or her primary domains of activity are planning, organizing, leading, and evaluating.

Nurse Practice Act. The basic enabling law in states and territories within the United States for licensure and definition of nursing practice in the jurisdiction of the legislative body establishing the act. It defines who may practice nursing and, to some extent, how nursing will be practiced in the jurisdiction.

nurses at every level. This phrase is used when it is important that direct-care nurses and nurses in every role, not solely nurse managers and nurse administrators, participate in decision-making bodies.

nurse satisfaction. Job satisfaction expressed by nurses working in hospital settings as determined by scaled responses to a uniform series of questions designed to elicit nursing staff attitudes toward specific aspects of their employment situation.

nursing research. A systematic search for knowledge about issues of importance to the nursing profession (Polit and Hungler, 1995).

nursing-sensitive indicators. "Measures and indicators that reflect the impact of nursing actions on outcomes" (American Nurses Association, 2004, p. 25).

organization. A stand-alone structure within an entity; the term can by used interchangeably with *setting* where appropriate or necessary.

outcomes. Quantitative and qualitative evidence related to the impact of structure and process on the patient, nursing workforce, organization, and consumer. These outcomes are dynamic; measurable; and may be reported at an individual unit, department, population, or organizational level. Donabedian (1980) defined *outcomes* as the "changes (desirable or undesirable) in individuals and populations that can be attributed to health care" (see 2003, p. 46).

patient. A healthcare consumer across the variety of settings; he or she might variously be called a *patient*, *client*, or *resident*.

patient falls. An unplanned descent to the floor, either with or without injury to the patient/resident/client. Calculated by the total number of patient falls times 1,000 divided by total number of patient days.

patient overall satisfaction. Patient opinion of the care received during the hospital stay as determined by scaled responses to a uniform series of questions designed to elicit patient views about global aspects of care.

patient satisfaction with educational information. Patient opinion of nursing staff efforts to educate about condition and care requirements as determined by scaled responses to a uniform series of questions designed to elicit patient views about specific aspects of education activities.

patient satisfaction with nursing care. Patient opinion of care received from nursing staff during the hospital stay as determined by scaled responses to a uniform series of questions designed to elicit patient views about components of nursing care services.

patient satisfaction with pain management. Patient opinion of how well nursing staff managed pain as determined by scaled responses to a uniform series of questions designed to elicit patient views about specific aspects of pain management.

peer evaluation. Peer-provided components of an annual evaluation or performance appraisal, which may or may not include peer review, by which registered nurses assess and judge the performance of professional peers (i.e., registered nurses with similar roles and education, clinical expertise, and level of licensure) against predetermined standards. The peer review process stimulates professionalism through increased accountability and promotes self-regulation of practice.

pressure ulcer occurrence. Any lesion caused by pressure resulting in damage of underlying tissues. Other terms used to indicate this condition include *bed sores* and *decubitus ulcers*.

pressure ulcer prevalence. Calculated as the total number of decubitus ulcers (Grade I–IV) times 1,000 divided by total number of patient days.

process. The actions involving the delivery of nursing and healthcare services to patients, including practices that are safe and ethical, autonomous, evidence-based, and focused on quality improvement. Donabedian (1980) defined process as the activities constituting health care, "including diagnosis, treatment, rehabilitation, prevention, and patient education—usually carried out by professional personnel, but also including other contributions to care, particularly by patients and their families" (see 2003, p. 46).

professional organization. Professional bodies, which may be known as *organizations*, *associations*, or *societies*, that usually have the purpose of advancing a profession and protecting the public interest. Many professional organizations include voluntary certification processes among their functions as a vehicle to verify that members meet certain prespecified standards.

professional practice model. The driving force of nursing care; a schematic description of a theory, phenomenon, or system that depicts how nurses practice, collaborate, communicate, and develop professionally to provide the highest quality care for those served by the organization (e.g., patients, families, community). Professional practice models illustrate the alignment and integration of nursing practice with the mission, vision, and values that nursing has adapted.

quality improvement (QI). "Systematic, data-guided activities designed to bring about immediate improvement in healthcare delivery in particular settings" (Lynn et al., 2007, p. 667).

registered nurse (RN). A nurse in the United States who holds state board licensure as a registered nurse or any new graduate or foreign nurse graduate who is awaiting state board examination results and is employed by a healthcare organization with responsibilities of an RN. In other countries, this individual will have registered with the appropriate regulatory body.

research. A systematic investigation, including research development, testing, and evaluation, designed to develop or contribute to generalizable knowledge. (U.S. Department of Health and Human Services, n.d., [45 CFR §46.102(d)] [21 CFR §50.3(k)] [21 CFR §312.3]). Research is distinguished from research utilization, the process of synthesizing, disseminating, and using research-generated knowledge to make an impact on, or a change in, the existing practices in society (Burns and Grove, 2005, p. 750).

setting. A stand-alone practice venue within an entity. The term can be used interchangeably with *facility* where appropriate or necessary.

shared leadership/participative decision-making. A model in which nurses are formally organized to make decisions about clinical practice standards, quality improvement, staff and professional development, and research.

staff nurse. A nurse whose primary responsibility is the provision of direct patient care (does not include clinical specialists).

standard. A norm that expresses an agreed-upon level of performance that has been developed to characterize, measure, and provide guidance for achieving excellence in practice.

strategic plan. A plan resulting from a process of "reviewing the mission, environmental surveillance, and previous planning decisions used to establish major goals and nonrecurring resource allocation decisions" (Griffith and White, 2002, p. 683).

structure. The characteristics of the organization and the healthcare system, including leadership, availability of resources, and professional practice models. Donabedian (1980) defined *structure* as the conditions under which care is provided, including material resources, human resources, and organizational characteristics "such as the organization of the medical and nursing staffs, the presence of teaching and research functions, kinds of supervision and performance review, and methods of paying for care" (see 2003, p. 46).

sufficient examples. Provided to indicate that compliance with a source of evidence is not isolated to a single group or area within the organization. While not every unit or clinical area must be represented, there should be evidence that the attribute exists throughout the breadth and depth of the organization.

system. A group of healthcare entities whose nursing is governed by a CNO as identified in this glossary and whether or not separately legally established as a for-profit or non-profit, corporation, association, sole proprietorship, or partnership.

transformational leadership. Leadership that identifies and communicates vision and values and asks for the involvement of the work group to achieve the vision (Burns, 1978, as cited in Dunham-Taylor, 2000).

turnover. Number of employees who resigned, retired, expired, or were terminated divided by the number employed during the same period.

vacancy rate. Calculated as 1 minus FTEs/WTEs employed divided by FTEs/WTEs budgeted times 100.